The Anti-Aging Diet Code

Newly Discovered Anti-Aging Diets
and Nutrition Guide That Makes
You Look 20-Years Younger

Dr. JERRY FUNG

DEDICATION

I will love to dedicate this book to the woman after my heart, my wife, and one true love. Thank you for your continuous love for me and our amazing children.

DISCLAIMER

In as much as i have written passionately and extensively on the matter, no part of this book should be taken as a legal or professional advice.

Take everything I have shared in this beautiful book as my opinion and regard it as a path to your own discoveries.

Please note that you are solely responsible for the actions you take by acting on the thoughts and views I shared in this book.

TABLE OF CONTENTS

Beautiful, bright skin begins with what we eat, but anti-aging foods may assist with so much more.

When we eat a diet rich in antioxidants, good fats, water, and necessary nutrients, our bodies express their gratitude through their greatest organ: our skin. After all, the skin is frequently the first area of our body to reveal signs of interior distress, and there are only so many lotions, creams, masks, and serums can do before we need to go deeper into our diets.

Many people spend their anti-aging efforts on expensive eye treatments, wrinkle-fighting serums, and even plastic surgery. While these things can certainly help, there is a more natural way to turn back the hands of time: eating your way to younger skin. Vitamin and mineral-rich foods can aid in the reversal of aging symptoms. The foods that include ellagic acid, biotin, and vitamins C and E, which are natural collagen boosters, are the greatest for your skin.

Researchers have even found that the safest and healthiest strategy to counteract dull complexions and fine lines is to consume fruits and vegetables. Are you ready to shine and turn the clock back?

Then stick with me as I reveal the Fountain of Youth's secrets and the Perfect Anti-Aging Diets that will make all the difference.

How Anti-Aging Treatments and Anti-Aging Diet Can Make You Feel 20 Years Younger

Anti-aging treatments are revolutionary breakthroughs! You can feel 10 to 20 years younger and discover a lifestyle full of energy and vitality by adding anti-aging nutrients and anti-aging supplements to your diet.

To be your best throughout your life, you should practice anti-aging tactics, use anti-aging treatments, eat well, and take supplements that will make you feel better and possibly even help you live longer. Chronological age does not always correspond to biological age. This is due to the fact that many people have mistreated their bodies in order to age faster than they need to. It can be outright misuse, such as drug and alcohol misuse, but more often than not, it is simply ignorance and a lack of correct anti-aging foods and supplements to help people stay healthy as they age.

You should exercise and consume a balanced diet to ensure that you stay as healthy as possible as you age. You can also use anti-aging treatments like special diet and anti-aging vitamins to help slow down the aging process. For example, certain vitamins and minerals battle free radicals, which assault your body's cells and speed up the aging process. As a result, your immune system is weakened, and you may become unwell. Anti-aging nutritional supplements can be bought at any health food store, as well as at your local department shop or on the internet.

Despite the fact that many of them are claimed to have significant benefits, you should see your doctor before taking any of them, since some of them may interact with any prescriptions you are now taking. To get the best results, look for natural anti-aging therapies and nutritional supplements that will help you avoid any negative side effects. Vitamin C and vitamin E are two examples of them. Green tea is also a powerful antioxidant beverage that can be used to replace at least some of your coffee consumption for improved health and vigor.

These compounds may help protect your body from certain malignancies and keep your heart healthy by helping to shield it from free radicals. These anti-aging treatments in the form of anti-aging nutritional supplements can assist fill in nutritional deficiencies that you may be experiencing in your diet, in addition to helping protect you against free radicals. While a result, as you develop your anti-aging and nutritional therapy plan, the supplements you take should include both vitamins and minerals such as calcium.

Diet, Nutrition, And Exercise That Can Help You Age Gracefully

Keep in mind that your anti-aging strategy should contain a variety of anti-aging treatments that work together to keep you healthy. To help you stay alive as you age, your anti-aging treatment strategy should involve both nutrition and activity. Because you'll be eating the correct meals with the right nutrition, including components that promote energy and contribute to antioxidant protection, you should notice an immediate boost in energy. A diet rich in anti-aging antioxidants, such as omega-3 fatty acids and plenty of fruits and vegetables, should be part of your anti-aging treatment strategy. Make every effort to eat only healthy, nutritional things in your diet.

Green leafy vegetables, barley grains, almonds, and extra-virgin olive oil are examples of these. These can improve your immune system and renew your cells. Organic vegetables have more nutrition and have not been cultivated with pesticides or other chemical residues that could end up in your food, so utilize them in your anti-aging treatment plan and diet whenever possible. These dietary adjustments can help reverse the aging process and lessen age-related adverse effects, in addition to simply making you feel better.

You should have more energy and enthusiasm for life. Refined flowers and sweets, as well as foods high in saturated and trans fats, are items to avoid in your diet for the optimum anti-aging effect. These meals cause your body to produce more free radicals and lack the nourishment you need to protect yourself from them. Keep in mind that for the greatest anti-aging treatment plan, you should combine your nutritional plan and food with a lifestyle that includes a healthy amount of physical exercise, as well as nutritional treatments and supplements.

Nutritional Foods For Anti-Aging Treatment

Fruits and veggies: When in doubt, choose colorful fruits and vegetables. For the maximum nutritional value and success in your anti-aging treatment plan, choose brightly colored fruits and vegetables that contain high levels of anti-aging antioxidants.

Fish: Fish high in omega-3 fatty acids, such as salmon, are good for your heart and brain, as well as providing other health advantages. If you don't like fish, you can take fish oil capsules instead. Some even have deodorizers in them, so you don't have to taste the fish if you don't like it. Other omega-3 fatty acids, such as flax oil, are a decent option if you are allergic to fish or can't eat it for whatever reason.

Yogurt: contains helpful bacterial enzymes, such as lactobacillus acidophilus, which are good bacteria that aid digestion.

Unsalted nuts: Unless you're allergic, eating little amounts of unsalted nuts every day (approximately 1 ounce) is ideal for optimal health. In your anti-aging therapy and nutritional diet, they contain both B vitamins and healthy fats that are essential for overall health.

Fiber: For maximum health, you should consume at least 25 grams of fiber each day, along with 8 ounces of water. This will assist you in staying regular and avoiding constipation. It will also make you feel fuller sooner, making you less prone to overeat.

Water: As previously said, you should drink at least 8 ounces of water every day. The water will not only aid digestion and relieve constipation, but it will also keep you fuller for longer, making you less prone to overeat. It also aids in the removal of toxins from your body, preventing them from remaining within your cells and speeding up the aging process.

Exercise and staying active, in addition to anti-aging treatments, will improve your health by strengthening strong muscles and providing adequate oxygen to your body cells, which will aid in the renewal of your entire body. Exercise is also an excellent technique to reduce weariness. People who are physically active have more energy to do normal duties and have more energy left over to enjoy other aspects of life.

Treatments For Anti-Aging Protection On The Skin

Despite your best efforts, your skin will eventually endure some changes as you age, such as wrinkling and sagging. However, by following a few simple steps to guarantee skin health, you may considerably slow down the rate at which this process occurs and possibly even reverse the consequences. The most important anti-aging skin treatment is to wear sunscreen whenever you are outside in the sun. The more fair your skin is, the greater your chance for skin cancer and other age-related aging disorders, such as age spots, wrinkles, and even skin cancer, depending on your family genetics. If you were exposed to a lot of unprotected sun as a child, you're also at danger. African-Americans have a built-in SPF of 300, making them the only ethnic group that may not require sunscreen, however lighter-skinned African-Americans may. In general, Caucasians require sunscreen, and the more protective the better. It should have a minimum of SPF 15 protection. This will help protect it from the harmful UV radiation that prematurely age skin and can even lead to skin cancer.

Furthermore, as you become older, certain anti-aging vitamins can help halt or even reverse the anti-aging process. Vitamins A, C, and E, for example, can help your skin regain its elasticity and give you a healthy shine. You could also want to try one of the new anti-aging therapies on the market, such as anti-aging or anti-wrinkle creams containing retinol, vitamin E, or Shea butter. Cocoa butter and coconut oil are two other helpful ingredients.

Of course, eating a balanced diet and drinking lots of water are the best things you can do for your skin. The nutrients and food provide your skin the nutrition it needs, and drinking plenty of water keeps pollutants from building up in your body. It will also aid in the hydration and appearance of your skin. Unfortunately, there is no miraculous anti-aging drug that will make you look or feel younger, but there are compounds that can help slow down the aging process, such as the vitamins and minerals mentioned earlier.

You have a higher chance of remaining bright well into your senior years if you follow these anti-aging treatment procedures, which include wearing sunscreen, exercising, eating a good diet, and drinking lots of water, as well as taking the supplements listed.

They should provide you greater energy and help you encounter fewer ailments as you age, so you may live your best life.

The Latest Anti-Aging Movement - The Pathway To The Fountain Of Youth

What is the significance of skincare in longevity research? I suppose a cell is a cell, and if you can unlock the code for one human cell, it's only a matter of time before you can crack the code for other sorts of cells - and the skin is without a doubt the most conspicuous cells we have. And it's our looks in particular that we frequently judge ourselves and others by, and we're inspected in turn, with opinions formed in a fraction of a second.

Our faces are often the first to exhibit symptoms of aging, and for many in modern culture, age is by definition "bad," and being young or appearing young is the ideal. That is why people invest billions of dollars each year on a variety of therapies aimed at reducing wrinkles, reversing the effects of gravity, and turning back the hands of time. With so much money at stake, many manufacturers are keen to find the next step in apprehending Father Time - or at the very least keeping him until the next stagecoach arrives, where he can perhaps be persuaded to go on before too much harm is done.

A friend once gave me a simple analogy that puts the whole situation in perspective. Although the research did not win a Nobel Prize, it provided me with the essential ah-ha moment.

The DNA strand's double helix - our most fundamental foundation for life - is held together at each end by things that act similarly to the hard plastic bits on the ends of shoelaces, preventing the DNA from unraveling and the individual chromosomes from scattering across the floor like a string of pearls down a marble staircase. Telomeres are the name for these structures.

The entire basis for how long the DNA stays intact is programmed somewhere into these small telomeres, and by implication, these are the keys to the organism's duration of life. A wonderful musical score is carved into the telomere, but like all musical scores, it has a double bar somewhere to indicate the conclusion; but is it a minuet or a Wagnerian epic? When the time comes for the telomeres to blow the full time whistle, the DNA strand will unravel and die, and the cycle of life will begin again. Telomeres control how often our skin cells are replaced, which explains why a puppy and a child born on the same day may appear to be the same age chronologically, but the dog has reached puberty before the child.

Telomeres, according to my buddy, occasionally go haywire (that must have a very specific scientific meaning). One way this happens is when they forget to release and unwind their programming, and instead just hang on, allowing the cells impacted to grow indefinitely without dying. In fact, when this happens frequently, they become exceedingly tough to destroy, and the cell - and those it propagates - is virtually immortal once the telomeres work in this way.

This ailment has a name that we are all familiar with. Cancer is a terrible disease.

But, if we could encourage the telomeres within a tumor to act normally in some way, wouldn't that be the "magic bullet" cure for cancer? Is this the recipe for a healthy cell that doesn't die if the telomeres in healthy cells can be taught to act like they do in cancer? Is this the only thread that holds the cure for cancer and immortality together?

Whatever your point of view, the reality is that some of the world's best research scientists are working on that precise subject, and some believe it will only be a decade or two until this is no longer speculation or science fiction, but a reality to confront. The societal changes that would occur even if life expectancy increased by 10 or 20 years would be huge, but we should all be considering this as a serious possibility.

From a dab of lanoline a generation ago to what I now hold in my hand as an anti-aging skincare treatment, it's been a revolution - and I'm confident that in a few years, I'll be saying that this cream will not only slow the aging process and reduce visible signs of aging, making your face appear younger - but it will actually be younger.

But first, let's take a look at how this whole quest for life extension and anti-aging began. Mankind has always aspired to immortality and fantasized about it, but the last 50 years have witnessed some significant progress toward this objective.

For millennia, mankind has pondered the possibility of extending life. The hunt for techniques to extend life can be traced all the way back to the Gilgamesh Epic.

Around 2500 BC, Gilgamesh was the fifth ruler of the kingdom of Uruk, which is now Iraq. He reigned for 126 years, according to the Sumerian list of monarchs. Methuselah lived nearly 900 years, according to the

Torah or Old Testament, with life spans estimated in centuries being uncommon before Noah's time.

Scholars have worked to solve this puzzle since the Reformation, and their efforts are still going strong today at the cutting edge of scientific research.

Secrets Revealed

We are beginning to comprehend what it is that causes us to grow from small babies to grownups as the secrets of our existence are unraveled in ever more minute detail. We now know, for example, that as the body ages, cell processes slow down and the creation of specific compounds needed by the body to rejuvenate decreases or stops entirely.

To keep its strength and stiffness, skin, for example, requires two components.

Collagen (strength and tightness) and elastin (flexibility) production declines as people get older. The reduction in production, combined with other variables such as the threat of free radicals, causes the skin to age and wrinkle. Free radicals are imperfect oxygen molecules that cause chain reactions within cells that are harmful.

Every cell, tissue, and organ in the human body goes through the same process. People get frown lines, crow's feet, and wrinkles, for example. Nutrients are no longer easily absorbed, and essential cell functions, hormones, and other chemicals are created at lower rates, causing the body to age.

A Historical Overview of the Life Extension Movement

For generations, scientists have been trying to find a way to slow down this process. However, it was not until around 1970 that life extension movements began to take shape.

Denham Harman, the founder of the so-called "free radical theory of aging," decided in this year that an organization dedicated to biogerontology (the branch of science concerned with the biological components of the aging process) study and information sharing was needed. The American Aging Association was founded as a result of this.

Philip Gordon and Joel Kurtzman, two futurists, published a book in 1976 on research towards extending human longevity. 'No More Dying' was the title of this popular collection. 'The Battle against Aging and the Extinction of Human Life.'

Kurtzman was then invited to testify before Florida's House Select Committee on Aging, which was chaired by Claude Pepper, an American politician and aging advocate. The purpose of this discussion was to discuss the implications of life extension on Social Security.

Saul Kent, a famous life extension activist, released the book 'The Life Extension Revolution' in 1980 and formed the nutraceutical (from 'nutrition' and 'pharmaceutical,' in other words, a nutrition supplement) company 'The Life Extension Foundation.'

This foundation is a non-profit that promotes dietary supplements and publishes the 'Life Extension Magazine' periodical. Kent later became active in cryogenics research. During the midst of this work, he was imprisoned for a dispute, but the charges were ultimately dropped.

With the book 'Life Extension: A Practical Scientific Approach,' published in 1982, American health writer and life extension advocate Sandy Shaw and her co-writer Durk Pearson popularized the phrase 'life extension' even more.

Another prominent book on the subject is 'Maximum Lifespan,' written by Roy Walford, a gerontologist and life-extensionist. In 1988, he and his student, Richard Weindruch, published a synopsis of the study they had done on the ability of calorie restriction to extend the life of mice. 'The Retardation of Aging and Disease by Dietary Restriction' is the title of this book.

Although the capacity to lengthen life by calorie restriction had been known since the 1930s, when gerontologist, biochemist, and nutritionist Clive McCay undertook some research into the matter, it was Walford and Weinbruch's work that offered substantial scientific footing to McCay's discoveries.

Walford's scientific effort was motivated by his personal desire to live longer. He lived a calorie-restricted lifestyle throughout his life and died at the age of 80. Amyotrophic lateral sclerosis, a progressive motor neuron disease, was the cause of his death.

The 'American Academy of Anti-Aging Medicine,' or A4M, was created in 1992 to establish an anti-aging medical specialty distinct from geriatrics. This enabled scientists and physicians interested in this topic to hold conferences and debate the most recent advancements.

Brian M. Delaney, a California-born author, philosopher, and translator, founded the sci.life-extension Usenet community. This was a significant step forward in the movement for life extension. The CR (Calorie Restriction) Society, for example, was founded as a result of it.

The idea of Dr. A. de Grey, a biogerontologist at Cambridge University, is a more recent development. This idea proposed that modern biotechnology may be used to restore damage to cells, macromolecules, organs, and tissues. For example, hair repair products demonstrate this.

Although it may appear that the majority of the work relating to life extension has been accomplished solely through the publication of books or the establishment of societies or organizations of some sort, the truth is that these books were written in response to or based on very specific, detailed scientific research that has yielded positive results.

They are no longer the creations of hopeful minds, but of determined scientists who have dedicated their life to learning more about aging and seeking to find ways to delay or even reverse the process.

Numerous discoveries have been made, and we are now able to extend lives to some extent in many ways. As a result of medical, pharmaceutical, and dietary breakthroughs brought about through research and development, the average lifespan of a human being is already significantly larger than it was previously.

The job goes on, and scientists all across the world are working on our behalf, conducting study, comparing data, discussing ideas, and making advancements.

What forces are propelling this push toward ever-increasing efforts to develop life-extension solutions? The answer to this issue is complicated by a number of things.

As the 'baby boomer' generation (those born between 1946 and 1964) approaches retirement age, their expectations are vastly different from those of previous generations. They have higher expectations and wishes to live life to the fullest as retirees for as long as feasible. This expectation encompasses not only length of life, but also quality of life, and it is frequently expressed as an active and vociferous demand rather than a quiet request.

Over the last two decades or more, advances in pharmacology have resulted in the development of a wide range of medications that allow people to live longer and more fulfilling lives. The research is currently ongoing, and new medications are being developed on a daily basis.

Erectile dysfunction medicines, such as Viagra, Cialis, and Levitra, are a classic example of a medicine that improves the quality of life for older people. These medications have significantly reduced the frequency of deaths and major injuries caused by old men rolling out of bed, as well as providing a number of other qualitative benefits.

Some recent scientific studies and subsequent developments in biotechnology and genetics are generating some optimism that some of the fundamental reasons of aging may be reversible.

As previously stated, chromosomes containing DNA strings are essentially capped with telomeres, a binding substance. In effect, telomeres are depleted during cell division, and they become shorter and shorter over time.

Leonard Hayflick was the first to notice this, and the mechanism of limiting cell proliferation was dubbed the Hayflick Limit after him. Advocates of life extension believe that by prolonging telomeres with medications or gene therapy, the Hayflick Limit may be extended and the cells, and hence the body, can be fooled into thinking it is younger than it is.

Nanotechnology, downsizing, computer chips, and robotics advancements also offer hope for potentially life-extending treatments.

In the 1970s, Lee Majors starred as the 'Six Million Dollar Man' on a popular TV show? Then it's science fiction. It is now scientifically proven. Millions of people today have artificial ankle, knee, and hip joints, as well as healthy feet. Mass manufacture of this technology was a pipe dream a generation ago.

Many people who have artificial limbs are in the same boat. The first artificial legs were primitive wooden contraptions that could only keep a person balanced. Artificial limbs are nearly entirely functioning nowadays.

Who would have guessed it would be able to bypass a coronary artery or perhaps replace a heart entirely 50 years ago? Hundreds of thousands, if not millions, of people are enjoying their lives as a result of this type of surgery, despite the fact that few of them would have been alive just half a century ago.

Because laser surgery is now available, millions of individuals no longer need to wear glasses. Only a few years ago, this, too, was science fiction. It is now advertised alongside shampoo in magazines and on television.

In other words, science is quickly progressing toward not only extending life but also improving the quality of those extra years.

What is it that the typical individual should believe? This is a question that is almost as tough to answer as figuring out how to live longer. Even among scientists, there are differing viewpoints. Some people believe that improving one's quality of life is as feasible as extending one's life span.

Others dismiss the idea as non-scientific gibberish. This is frequently motivated by a fear of anything 'new' upsetting the status quo of established boundaries. Fortunately, real scientists keep looking, since if every scientist determined that any of the current medical, pharmaceutical, and technological advances could not be made, we would all be dead by the age of 30.

There is no doubt that there are a lot of charlatans out there trying to make a quick buck off people's desire to stay young. Many goods sold in the millions nowadays are fundamentally ineffective; they are often given spectacular names and contain the most perplexing chemicals to make them appear scientific to consumers and justify their cost.

However, while numerous advances are being made and research indicates to the prospect of one day discovering the key to staying young for longer, the scientific community continues to warn the public that many of the products on the market today are unreliable to say the least.

Although food supplements may help to keep a body healthier - something that can often be accomplished simply by adopting a healthy lifestyle and diet - there is no categorical and unequivocal proof that they actually slow down aging.

Many hormone therapies are the same way. Although they may have a short-term effect, they have yet to be scientifically demonstrated to be effective in the long run. The concern that it might not work stems from the fact that taking hormones, such as those used in hormonal acne treatment, slows down the body's own production of these hormones.

Furthermore, many treatments may have long-term (but undiscovered) negative effects that are hazardous to the user's health. There are concerns that hormone therapies may increase the risk of cancer, diabetes, and other serious conditions.

Other approaches, such as calorie restriction, have proven to be effective in rodents. In fact, tests with rats on limited diets of 30 to 50 percent have shown that they can practically double their lifespan.

Similar research on primates has revealed a tendency to extend life and protect against a variety of age-related disorders. Human studies have yet to be conducted, despite the fact that some people do follow calorie-restricted diets. However, whether or not this will help them live longer is something that will have to be seen.

According to the hypothesis, lowering calorie consumption slows the body's metabolism, which in turn slows the aging process. According to nutritionists, a body of a specific size and weight requires a particular number of calories to stay healthy. In the long run, cutting this amount by up to 50% is not a good idea.

As they say, only time will tell, but how will anyone know the difference? Is it because a person is on this diet that they live to the age of 80, or would they have lived to this age anyway?

Many people feel that major progress in the field of longevity can be expected during the next two decades. This group generally believes that genetics and biotechnology will finally provide the answer. It's too early to make firm predictions, but the study so far has shown promise, and some of the findings are already being applied in particular treatments to improve patients' lives, as noted previously.

To say the least, overall aging is impossible to slow down at the moment. Some products claim to help with overall health and longevity, but the first commercial products are currently being produced in the area of skin care, and given the magnitude of this market, it is probable that this will continue to be the weather-vane of longevity treatments.

For many years, it will be difficult to tell these two apart. Because it is difficult to disprove many theories, charlatans are likely to exist. Positive proof from those on the trail of a real breakthrough with an ethical perspective will be equally tough, as items based on solid research and using technology or chemicals that will genuinely have an effect rarely claim instant results. This is something that anyone aiming for more youthful appearances, for example, should keep in mind. None of these items are capable of performing miracles. Even the best of them will require time and consistent use to attain the desired result.

The bottom line is that, as things stand now, we can be certain that certain things are ineffectual or even harmful; others show promise; and still others are beginning to cross the threshold into being able to produce outcomes - if marginally.

Meanwhile, it's a good idea to do a lot of research on products and avoid being fooled by strange and wonderful-sounding substances or fantastic-sounding promises of instant youth. Regeneration will take time - let's face it, it's taken a lifetime to get here, and there's no way to turn back the clock in an instant.

One would wonder what all of this, especially the life extension movement as a whole, has to do with skin care, health, and beauty goods. As a result of much of the study into life extension, new approaches to skin care are emerging as a by-product.

These research and development teams can explore new substances, their compatibility with human cells, and genetic make-up, thanks to a better understanding of how genetics and cellular processes affect skin aging and condition.

Many substances found in nature are not only compatible with human skin, but they also have natural receptors in the skin cells. Because these receptors have been found as a result of life extension research, skin care companies may now use this information to formulate products that have the greatest impact.

The use of nanotechnology is another 'by-product' of life extension research in terms of skin care. The use of nanotechnology, or more precisely, nanoparticles, has had a significant impact on the delivery of nutrients and other ingredients in skin care products to skin cells. Nanotechnology has already revolutionized skin care in certain ways. It's now feasible to use active compounds that were previously difficult to transport to the skin, as well as improve the efficacy of tried-and-true compounds. Some cosmetic chemicals that have been used in some cultures for hundreds, if not thousands of years can today be employed even more effectively to improve skin condition and preserve a healthy, youthful appearance.

Nanotechnology can even boost the hydrating impact of skin care products. Nanosomes are employed to achieve this effect. Nanosomes are tiny, pocket-like particles that melt or disintegrate when they come into touch with the skin. The moisturizing impact is hastened as a result, aiding the skin faster and more effectively.

Nanotechnology is thought to play a role in not just reducing the aging of skin, but also in repairing and mending skin cells and tissue.

The study of stem cells is another accomplishment in life extension research that is beginning to show up in skin care products. Stem cells are found in all forms of life, including plants, animals, and humans. Other cells lack two characteristics that stem cells possess. The ability to develop into any cell type and the ability to divide practically endlessly are two of these traits. The use of plant stem cell extracts in skin care is expected to be one of the industry's next "great things." And brace yourself for the uproar if human stem cells are recommended as part of an anti-aging skincare regimen, which will undoubtedly happen!

One thing is certain: science will continue to seek answers to the topic of life extension, and business will drive the commercialization of breakthroughs. But whether these lead to a utopian future or a minefield of conflict as we argue who will utilize and benefit from these new godlike capabilities remains to be seen. Meanwhile, on a practical level, in the skincare, health, and beauty industries, we remain hopeful and anticipating that solutions will emerge that not only promise but provide benefits.

The Best Anti-Ageing Drinks For Women To Look Smashing Young

Every woman wishes to appear and remain youthful for as long as feasible. To keep your age at bay, you experiment with various cosmetic items. However, you should be aware that cosmetics are not the sole means of combating ageing effects. Cosmetics, on the other hand, contain chemicals and preservatives that might harm your skin. To achieve younger-looking soft, supple skin, women must keep a healthy lifestyle and eat a balanced diet. If you can maintain a healthy lifestyle, you will have good health on the inside and out. You may improve your beauty and keep it for longer by doing workouts or engaging in any type of activity such as dancing, playing, or swimming. People who are too busy to spend time to such activities can practice yoga at home. Yoga is an excellent strategy to keep your youth. The most crucial is fluid intake, which has numerous health benefits and helps you stay active and youthful. Here are the top ten drinks for staying youthful.

• Drink plenty of water – an adult should drink at least 2-3 liters of water per day (no more unless suggested by a doctor) to keep their system clean. The best method to stay young is to drink enough of water. The organs will function properly and you will stay hydrated throughout the day if you drink enough water. Hydrated cells are more elastic, and more elasticity implies less wrinkles, which translates to skin that seems to be younger.

• Drink Green Tea - Green tea contains polyphenols, which assist to slow down the aging process. Green tea use on a regular basis can help you see a difference in just a few days. Green tea detoxifies your body by draining out all impurities and is one of the finest sources of Catechins, which protect cells from free radical-induced oxidation. Free radicals are known to cause cell damage, which can lead to a variety of health issues, including premature aging.

• Choose Appropriate Alcohol - Certain types of alcohol can help you stay young. Alcohol consumption in moderation increases brain cell activity, which aids in the prevention of aging. Red wine, for example, contains grape juice extracts, making it the most popular and useful drink for women looking to regain their youthful glow.

• Drink Carrot Juice on a Regular Basis - Carrots include flavonoids, which are antioxidants that help to kill free radicals. Free radicals are damaging to our health and have been linked to a variety of illnesses, including accelerated aging.

• Soy Milk Isn't a Milk Substitute - Lactose intolerance is common among women, so they drink soy milk. However, soy milk is the most effective anti-aging beverage among the top ten drinks for women. Flavones are a component that helps to maintain collagen levels and prevent collagen breakdown. These practical exercises help you obtain firmer skin, slow the aging process, and keep your skin's youthful texture and gloss. As a result, if you want to stay young for a long time, you should include soy milk in your normal diet.

• Cocoa drinks have anti-aging properties for ladies - Flavones are unique components found in cocoa, according to experts. It aids in the improvement of blood circulation, focus, and flow. Flavones are an important component that aids in the smooth functioning of the body and the restoration of the lost glow that occurs as a result of the aging process. This allows your system to function properly, allowing you to stay young and healthy.

• The Beneficial Beetroot Juice—daily use of beetroot juice improves blood flow to the brain and alleviates age-related issues such as dementia. Nitrate, which is found in beets, has anti-aging benefits. The huge amount of nitrate gives you the ability to combat the aging process. To live a longer life, include cabbages, radishes, and other green vegetables in your diet. Vegetable smoothies can be substituted for juice.

• Drinking a cup of coffee has numerous health benefits. Almost everyone enjoys a cup of coffee. Coffee contains polynoids, which help you fight skin cancer, Alzheimer's disease, and Parkinson's disease, as well as keep you from becoming old.

• Drinking milk: Milk is high in vitamins, minerals, proteins, calcium, and other nutrients. Milk helps to protect your bones, teeth, blood pressure, and cardiovascular health. Adults should have 800 milligrams of milk each day, while teenagers should have 100 milligrams.

Pomegranate, Orange, or Lemon Juice - Fruits are high in fiber, vitamins, minerals, and antioxidants. Each fruit has its own distinct characteristics. You should drink a variety of fruit juices on a daily basis. Some specific fruits contain anti-aging characteristics and aid in the battle against ageing influences. Pomegranate, orange, grapefruit, gooseberry, lemon, and other fruits fall into this category. Fruits are high in vitamin C and antioxidants, which assist to slow down the aging process and maintain a young appearance.

You can stay young, healthy, fit, and active in a variety of ways, regardless of your gender or age. Every day, after you wake up, drink one glass of warm water with lemon juice and honey. This drink will assist you in eliminating all pollutants and toxins from your body. It's widely used for detoxification. Your system will remain renewed throughout the process if these early ageing triggers are removed. You can improve your results by drinking some medicinal plant juice. Basil leaves, Neem leaves, and turmeric juice, for example, can be quite beneficial to your health. The antiseptic and antibacterial qualities of neem, basil, and turmeric encourage the formation of skin cells, resulting in healthy skin and a youthful appearance.

The top ten drinks for women to stay young and healthy have been thoroughly reviewed in order to provide you a better understanding of the advantages of choosing natural organic beverages to live a healthier and more fulfilling life. If you follow these instructions and avoid processed drinks and foods, you will find all of the above recommendations to be beneficial. After receiving a comprehensive health exam under expert supervision, you can follow these guidelines. Remember to follow the instructions, and you can simply slow down the aging process by drinking more water.

Present and Future Anti-Aging Treatments and Diets – A view At Anti-Oxidants

The study of the anti-aging effects of anti-oxidants in the recent years has left scientists and nutritionists surprised as the possibility of retaining youth, just by eating more of the diets we neglect. Vitamin C and E, for example, are natural anti-oxidants that function together. Antioxidants from a diet rich in fruits and vegetables may be more effective. Antioxidant-rich fruits and vegetables should be consumed in 6 or more servings each day, according to nutritionists. Although everyone believes that taking antioxidant supplements for anti-aging can be beneficial, there is no consensus on the most effective supplement amounts.

Anti-aging medicine recognizes that stress of any kind accelerates the aging process, but it has yet to find a tailored treatment for it. Internal and environmental stressors abound, and individual stress levels vary significantly. Improper hydration is an often-overlooked source of internal tension. Water is required for the proper functioning of numerous physiological functions. Water deficiency or excess promotes age-related stress. Thirst perception declines with age (80+), and dehydration can readily develop in. Antioxidants are another source of stress that is often underestimated. Supplemental anti-oxidants in high dosages (or doses above specific but defined quantities) are known to cause stress.

Antioxidant supplements must prevent other types of stress in addition to the stress they cause to be effective. Knowing the proper supplement amounts to do this is an important aspect of anti-aging treatment. Internal tension is lower in a healthy young guy in his twenties who is properly nourished than in an older person in his sixties. Lower antioxidant doses may be safer for a young person than higher doses. Higher doses of antioxidants may aid an elderly person whose many internal homeostatic processes are less capable of dealing with internal stress. A course of anti-ageing treatment based on antioxidants should theoretically lower the rate at which cellular damage occurs. The rate at which cells become "sick" will slow down. The number of cells with longer telomere chains will increase with time as fewer diseased cells are replaced at a slower pace. As a result, you might reasonably expect an increase in life expectancy. For now, increasing your daily diet of anti-oxidant-rich fruits and vegetables, slightly increasing your antioxidant consumption, and taking various vitamins and modest amounts of anti-aging supplements on a daily basis is the recommended but imprecise method to slowing the pace of cellular damage. According to one study, taking a high-quality multivitamin supplement is linked to greater telomere length.

Anti-aging treatment should ideally be tailored to each individual. On an individual basis, the goal would be to measure and limit the cumulative impacts of various types of stress. Practical biomarkers for various types of stress that are easily measured do not yet exist or are not being employed. It will be simple to modify individual antioxidant dosages once they are in use, ensuring that everyone has "optimum" amounts throughout their lives. The body would have a safe store of protecting antioxidants at "optimal" levels.

Following that, I'll go over the most common nutrients linked to anti-aging. Beta-carotene (vitamin A), vitamin C, vitamin E, different flavonoids, omega-3 and omega-6 fatty acids, Co-enzyme Q10, Lycopene, and Selenium are some of the most well-known anti-oxidants, vitamins, and nutrients linked to good health and anti-aging.

There are a slew of supplements that have been shown to effectively cure certain aging symptoms. DMAE,

Acetyl-l-carnitine, L-carnosine, Alpha Lipoic Acid, DHEA, L-arginine, and melatonin are a few of the more well-known supplements.

Some of the anti-oxidants described before can be found in good meals. Green Tea, turmeric, and red wine are a few more notable foods linked to anti-aging.

All of the aforementioned have distinct biological features and, in my opinion, are "healthy" for you when consumed in small or moderate doses. Some (for example, vitamin C) may be "beneficial" for you in higher doses. Various studies on any of these subjects may contradict one another. You'll have to do your own research on each ingredient, but experts have already discovered that some foods are linked to telomere lengths that are longer than typical. Green Tea, Omega-3, Vitamins A, C, D, and E are among them.

- Vitamin E has been linked to anti-aging telomere lengthening effects.
- Green tea is high in antioxidants such as vitamin C, vitamin E, and flavonoids.
- Flavonoids (which include catechins and quercetin) are a type of antioxidant that possesses anticarcinogenic, antihypercholesterolemic, antibacterial (which helps prevent dental caries),

and anti-inflammatory activities. Polyphenols abound in the tea plant's leaves. Green tea consumption of three cups or more per day has been linked to telomere lengths that are longer than norm.

- Omega-3 fatty acids are anti-inflammatory long-chain polyunsaturated fatty acids that help prevent heart disease, stroke, memory loss, depression, arthritis, cataracts, and cancer. Omega-3 fatty acids prevent the shortening of telomeres, which may prevent cells from aging.

Vitamin C is a water-soluble antioxidant found throughout the body that protects cellular components from free radical production caused by pollution and cigarette smoke. Many studies have linked high vitamin C intake to a lower risk of mouth, laryngeal, and esophageal cancer. Vitamin C has showed promise in the treatment of premature aging, as well as the prevention of aging.

I was unable to provide further reference links to support the preceding paragraphs due to constraints on the amount of links I could include in this post. If you're interested, please email me at the address listed at the bottom of this page and I'll send them to you.

The sooner you begin an anti-aging treatment, the better; however, it is never too late to begin. All genuine treatments will assist you in maintaining a telomere chain length that is longer than the average.

The programmed death theory of aging aims to address the underlying causes of aging. Attempts to halt or reverse the telomere shortening process are part of this quest. TA 65 and human genetic engineering are two such medicines.

Sierra Sciences manufactures and markets TA 65, a telomerase activator. Astragalus, a plant extract with telomerase activation characteristics, is the main element in TA 65. Although the product may be effective, I do not endorse it for a variety of reasons. For the typical person, TA 65 is prohibitively pricey. TA 65 is used in the programs of a number of high-end health spas. These are, once again, financially out of reach of the typical person. Many people have questioned Sierra Sciences' marketing techniques, and there are lawsuits ongoing against TA 65.

The main problem I have with TA 65 is that it is not scientifically honest. The business created genetically modified mice that could switch telomerase on and off at a young age. TA 65 was able to reactivate telomerase in these mice, allowing them to resume their usual lives.

It is dishonest to use this to demonstrate the efficacy of the TA65 treatment. This is not how telomerase normally functions, and the lifetime was not extended beyond what it would have been without the genetic change. The effects of TA65 on normal mice were transient, with little or no life extension.

The real key to combating and conquering aging is human genetic engineering. It has the potential to directly address the causes of aging. CRISPR, for example, allows DNA base pairs to be inserted or removed at particular locations in our DNA. As a result, the human genome can now be fine-tuned as needed. Telomerase gene therapy has been shown to extend the longevity of aged mice. In humans, gene modification therapy has been utilized to treat a variety of medical issues. Elizabeth Parrish became the first human to get anti-aging gene therapy on September 15, 2015. As our understanding of the specifics of the human genome expands, anti-aging medicines will swiftly progress.

Current social and political attitudes seem to encourage the advancement of anti-aging research. Although there are no internationally recognized political initiatives to stop aging or lengthen life, a few pro-immortality political parties have emerged since 2012. Their mission is to encourage anti-aging and life extension research, as well as to ensure that everyone has access to developments in these fields. The SENS (Strategies for Engineered Negligible Senescence) organization, which is one of the many organizations sponsoring anti-aging research, has devised an anti-aging research strategy. They hope to create anti-aging treatments that can restore a wide range of cellular damage. SENS is a non-profit organization. Any anti-aging breakthroughs made possible by the financing it gives will be widely publicized. Aside from conventional scientific study, the Palo Alto Longevity Prize of $1,000,00 is being awarded to anyone who can develop a successful anti-aging medication.

All known anti-aging medications are only half successful as of 2015. One can definitely extend one's life by 10 to 25 years depending on when one begins a complete anti-aging program. An anti-aging lifestyle, according to Harvard School of Public Health researchers, can add 24.6 extra productive years to one's lifespan. Every ten years, anti-aging knowledge increases by around tenfold. This most likely means that many of us have plenty of time to reap the anticipated advantages of anti-aging science. Aging, like many other disorders, will be cured one day. While we wait for those anti-aging technological singularity to arrive, the goal is to stay healthy long enough to reap the benefits.

How to Prepare the perfect Anti-Aging Breakfast

Breakfast is said to be the most important meal of the day. A nutritious breakfast is not only good for you, but it may also help you live longer. While everyone grows older, starting your day with nutrient-dense foods, such as one or more servings of fruits and vegetables high in anti-aging nutrients such as vitamin C, may help you live longer. You can also include a lean source of protein and whole grains that are proven to combat aging, such as oatmeal.

Method No. 1:

Including Fruits and Vegetables in Your Diet

Make yourself a green smoothie. Greens such as kale and spinach are high in vitamins and minerals, making them an excellent smoothie base. Greens are high in B vitamins and fiber, which can help you fight the indications of aging and avoid degenerative diseases. Blend one cup of greens with one cup of water, then add two cups of fruit to the blender.

Green smoothies with spinach, pineapple, and mango are delicious.

Combine kale, strawberries, and pineapple in a green smoothie.

Take a bite of an orange. If you're in a rush, grab an orange for an anti-aging breakfast on the fly. Oranges are high in vitamin C and help moisturize skin and tissues. Vitamin C can assist your body in producing collagen more effectively.

For an anti-aging boost, start your day with a glass of orange juice.

As part of a portable breakfast, bring an orange to work. To keep natural sugars to a minimum, keep the size to 4 oz.

Add some avocado to the mix. This fruit is high in monounsaturated fat, which can help your skin stay hydrated. Avocado is a great anti-aging breakfast because monounsaturated fats help your body absorb nutrients from other foods.

Serve with half a grapefruit and a slice of avocado on whole grain bread.

Avocado is a great way to add healthy fats to your green smoothie.

Take a pomegranate and eat it. Pomegranates are high in nutrients that can help counteract the effects of aging. High cholesterol, high blood pressure, and inflammatory illness can all be treated and even prevented with this fruit. Pomegranates have also been demonstrated to lower the likelihood of heart disease risk factors.

To a breakfast of turkey bacon and avocado toast, add a glass of pomegranate juice.

Pomegranate juice can be added to a smoothie or a bowl of oatmeal to give it a boost.

Take a grapefruit and eat it. Grapefruit can help lower "bad" cholesterol while increasing "good" cholesterol levels in the body. Grapefruit has also been related to weight loss and decreased insulin resistance, so it's a great anti-aging breakfast option.

Some medications, such as Warfarin, can interact with grapefruit. Consult your doctor to ensure that eating or drinking grapefruit is safe for you.

For breakfast, try half a grapefruit with some lean protein, such as chicken breakfast sausage.

A glass of grapefruit juice can be added to any breakfast for an anti-aging vitamin C boost.

Breakfast should include blueberries. Micronutrients abound in this small fruit. Blueberry-rich diets have been related to increased motor skills and memory, as well as a lower risk of heart attack and cholesterol. As part of an anti-aging breakfast, consume one cup (15 grams) of blueberries three to four times a week.

For a quick and easy breakfast, combine a handful of blueberries with a small bowl of Greek yogurt.

For a quick breakfast, grab a whole-grain blueberry muffin.

Method No. 2:

Including Whole Grains and Healthy Proteins

Choose protein sources that are low in fat. A lean protein source should be part of your anti-aging breakfast. High-fat protein sources can cause inflammation, which can speed up the aging process. You can use turkey bacon or chicken sausage as lean meat sources. Lentils, beans, tofu, and dairy are all good sources of protein for breakfast.

Breakfast may be a cup of last night's lentil stew if you think outside the cereal box.

Consume an egg. This morning classic is high in B vitamins, which can help with memory and cognitive function. Lutein is also found in eggs, and it can help prevent against vision loss as you get older.

Top a toasted whole grain English muffin with an egg and sliced avocado.

Scrambled eggs go well with fruit or a green smoothie.

Add a handful of nuts to the mix. Nuts are always a terrific addition and healthy source of nutrients, no matter what you choose to make for an anti-aging breakfast. Healthy fats, proteins, vitamins, minerals, and antioxidants abound in nuts. They're also available in a range of colors.

Nuts are delicious when eaten by the handful. Toss a handful of almonds on top of a fruit and yogurt bowl. On your way out the door, grab a single-serving bag of unsalted almonds, walnuts, pistachios, cashews, or pecans for a light anti-aging breakfast.

Nut butters are also a wonderful option. Consider spreading natural almond, peanut, or cashew butter on whole grain toast or on fruit, as raw nuts often provide more advantages than store-bought peanut butter (particularly with added sugar and salt). Nut butter is especially beneficial for senior persons who have difficulty chewing.

Make yourself a dish of oats. Soluble fiber is abundant in oats, which can aid in the reduction of "bad" cholesterol. Antioxidants included in oats may help prevent cell damage, decrease fine lines and wrinkles, and make your skin look plumper. Oats are also low-glycemic, meaning they won't produce a blood sugar increase.

For a quick anti-aging breakfast, toss a handful of your favorite fruit into a bowl of oatmeal.

Simple Anti-Aging Diet And Lifestyle Tips That Reverse Your Age

It's difficult to predict how the aging process will affect you until it happens to you. Then one morning, as you get out of bed, your knees begin to hurt, your brow develops lines the size of Whole Foods on a Sunday afternoon, and that cup of coffee you just made vanishes into the ether—along with your car keys.

You wish you could go back in time right now.

While scientists may be years (or, more likely, an eternity) away from understanding how to stop time in its tracks, exercising better habits in your own life can have a significant impact on how you age. Our anti-aging secrets for a younger you will have your pals yearning to know how you've turned back the clock, from preventing skin damage to extending your life expectancy. Add these 40 Best-Ever Fat-Burning Foods to your meal when you're ready to take your healthy living strategy to the next level.

1. Reduce your weight

Losing weight is often at the top of our yearly resolutions list, but getting started on it sooner rather than later could give you more years to look forward to. Obesity is linked to a higher risk of heart disease, embolisms, diabetes, and certain types of cancer, according to research published in the American Journal of Clinical Nutrition, and carrying additional pounds can deplete your vitality in an instant. Fortunately, research shows that decreasing just 10% of your total body weight can significantly improve your life expectancy and overall health.

2. Bananas are a great snack

Snacking on a banana is one fountain of youth advice that's as simple as it is a-peeling. Bananas are high in potassium, which can help your heart stay healthy and minimize muscle cramps, making it simpler to go to the gym every day. Even better, researchers from Lund University in Sweden have connected resistant starch in foods like bananas to healthier gut bacteria, which can lower your risk of Alzheimer's disease.

3. Dance is a great way to express yourself

Even if you're not quite the dancing with the Stars material, busting a move might be beneficial to your health, especially as you become older. Senior citizens who attended dance lessons three times a week had more density in the areas of their brain linked with memory and information processing than those who were sedentary or went on walks for exercise, according to research published in Frontiers in Aging Neuroscience.

4. Include green vegetables in every meal

While our food pyramid suggests that grains should make up the majority of our diets, greens can help us stay healthier for longer. Increased consumption of leafy greens is connected to lower incidence of Alzheimer's disease and other indicators of brain aging, according to research published in Alzheimer's & Dementia. All those antioxidants you'll be adding to your meal with every cup of kale or spinach salad can help your skin stay healthy and glowing.

5. Scrambled Eggs Are A Great Way To Begin Your Day

Switching from carb-heavy breakfasts to eggs is an eggcellent approach to slow down the aging process. Researchers at the University of Wisconsin discovered that the combination of lutein and zeaxanthin present in egg yolks can help prevent macular degeneration, keeping your eyes clean and healthy as you get older. According to the findings of a study published in the

International Journal of Obesity, those who ate eggs for breakfast lost considerably more weight than those who ate bagels for breakfast.

6. Consume Grapes

Choosing red grapes over your typical sweet treat could make you look and feel years younger in no time. Red grapes are high in resveratrol, an antioxidant that can help you lose belly fat and has been related to increased eye circulation, which can help you keep your vision sharp as you age, according to a study conducted at Washington University School of Medicine.

7. Emphasize the positive aspects of life

A little optimistic thinking might go a long way toward helping you turn back the clock.

According to research published in the Journal of Personality and Social Psychology, elderly nuns who had positive things to say about their lives had a lower chance of dying, and looking on the bright side can also make you appear younger.

8. Vitamin C should be consumed in large quantities

Increasing your vitamin C consumption with fresh citrus fruit will have all of your pals wondering what you've done to look years younger. According to a study published in the International Journal of Cosmetic Science, vitamin C can boost your body's collagen production and skin firmness, preventing cellulite and sagging. However, adding citrus to your diet will benefit more than just your appearance; researchers in Bordeaux discovered a link between citrus flavonoid consumption and reduced cognitive decline, and studies have even linked high vitamin C levels to reduced stress and better sleep, all of which can help you look younger.

9. Apricots Should Be in Your Menu

All it takes is a quick snack to turn back the clock. If you eat a few dried apricots instead of a preservative-laden convenience meal, you might be able to keep your youthful vigor. Apricots are high in beta-carotene, which has been linked to a lower risk of Alzheimer's disease and other forms of cognitive decline by researchers at Ulm University in Germany. Apricots also include a powerful mixture of vitamins A, C, and E, which has been demonstrated to help prevent age-related eye problems. Just make sure your apricots are free of added sugar, which can age your skin, and sulfite preservatives, which are a major cause of allergic reactions.

10. Reduce your calorie intake

Dieting isn't always enjoyable, but it has the potential to improve your health and life. Losing weight not only lowers your risk of a variety of chronic diseases, but UCLA researchers discovered that mice that lowered their caloric load by 65 percent lived 35 to 65 percent longer than mice that had modest caloric restriction. They were also able to reduce their chances of developing a tumor.

11th. Soup made with butternut squash

Are you looking for some delicious comfort food? Instead of reaching for fried or sugary foods that can hasten your aging process, make a bowl of butternut squash soup. Butternut squash is high in beta-carotene, which has been shown to decrease the pace of noticeable skin aging in a research published in Dermato Endocrinology.

12. Inventive+ phrasing Blueberries as a Snack

No matter your age, tossing some blueberries into your oatmeal or favorite smoothie can help you preserve your young glow. Anthocyanins, the antioxidant pigments that give blueberries their unique color, greatly reduce the risk of dementia in the aging brain, according to research published in the Annals of the New York Academy of Sciences.

13th. Dark Chocolate should be consumed

Is there a way to slow down the aging process? A small amount of dark chocolate is one hell of a trick to do just that. Dark chocolate's caffeine can help you feel energized, and research suggests that it can raise serotonin levels in your brain. Researchers at the Witten/Herdecke Institute for Experimental Dermatology have even linked cocoa flavonols to reduced sun damage risk, keeping your skin looking as young as it did when you were a teenager.

14th. A Constant Sprinkling of sesame seeds

That sesame-crusted tuna you had for supper the other night might just be your best barrier against the effects of aging. Sesame seeds are a strong source of calcium that fights osteoporosis, with 88 milligrams per tablespoon, lessening your chance of fractures and early mortality every time you consume them. Do you think a glass of milk or a slice of cheese will provide the same benefit? Reconsider your position. According to the findings of a study published in the BMJ, dairy can speed up bone demineralization and raise your risk of osteoporosis.

15th. Make Asparagus a Part of Your Menu

Get your gut health in tip-top shape, and you might just be able to turn back the clock. Because your gut contains 70% of your immune system, it's critical to keep the delicate balance of bacteria in your stomach in order to avoid significant health problems; in fact, research from Lund University in Sweden has connected healthy belly bacteria to a lower risk of Alzheimer's disease. Fortunately, adding some asparagus to your diet could be all you need to improve your gut health. Asparagus is high in inulin, a prebiotic fiber that nourishes your gut flora, allowing them to support your immune system.

16. Increase Your Fiber Consumption

Increasing your fiber intake could be the first step toward a more youthful appearance. Consuming fiber-rich foods can aid in the growth of beneficial gut bacteria, increasing your immune system and lowering your risk of illness. High-fiber diets have also been linked to a lower risk of colon cancer and can help you get rid of that bloated stomach that makes you seem years older than you are.

17th. Make Brussels Sprouts a Regular Part of Your Diet

Do you want to appear younger? Let's get the Brussels sprouts going. Brussels sprouts are high in lutein, which has been related to a reduction in UV damage and skin cancer in studies conducted at Georgian Court University. Lutein can also help prevent the loss of natural elastin in your skin, which keeps you appearing young by preventing fine lines and wrinkles.

18. Do Some Endurance Workouts

A little endurance exercise may be just what you need to feel healthier, more energized, and younger. Endurance training can lower inflammation and help retain skeletal muscle even as you get older, keeping you strong and avoiding the skin-sagging effects of muscle loss, according to research published in Mechanisms of Ageing and Development.

How To Use Vitamin C To Prepare Your Own Anti-Aging Body Lotions And Creams

Vitamin C is well-known for its immune-boosting properties. It is, nevertheless, an important nutrient that aids in the formation of collagen. Vitamin C and collagen help to revitalize the skin by repairing damaged cells and restoring firmness and suppleness. Using one of the two ways below, you may make your own vitamin C anti-aging lotion at home quickly and easily.

1st method:

Using Glycerin from Vegetables

Using distilled water, dissolve vitamin C powder. In a small container, combine 12 teaspoon vitamin C powder with 1 tablespoon (14.8 ml) purified water. To avoid a gritty mixture, mix the components together until the powder is completely dissolved.

Use only distilled water, not filtered or unfiltered tap water.

This is due to the high oxygen levels in tap water, which allows the components to break down more quickly.

Last in mind that your water and vitamin C mixture will only keep for two weeks in the refrigerator, after which time the serum should be discarded.

Glycerin should be added to the vitamin C combination. The purpose of glycerin is to smooth out the solution and hydrate the skin. 2 tbsp vegetable glycerin (29.6 ml) If you used glycerin in the first batch, you should use less water in the second batch.

In this situation, instead of 1 tablespoon (14.8 ml), 1 teaspoon of distilled water will be added to the mixture.

When glycerin is added, the mixture will last for a month.

Fill an amber apothecary container halfway with serum. Now your vitamin C cream is ready to be stored. Put it in the fridge to keep it fresh and prevent it from breaking down.

Because exposing vitamin C to light reduces its efficacy and causes it to oxidize fast, making it less effective, darker bottles are preferable.

2nd Method

Using Almond Oil as a Base

Make a vitamin C and distilled water mixture. In a glass jar, combine 12 teaspoon vitamin C and 5 teaspoons purified water. Because vitamin C takes time to dissolve, mix it thoroughly.

It should be stirred repeatedly until it is completely dissolved, with no gritty particles remaining in the liquid.

Toss in 3 teaspoons almond oil into the mix. Almond oil advantages include sun protection, rejuvenation and softness of the skin, and reduction of scars, inflammation, and skin irritation.

Almond oil is high in vitamins A, B, and E, all of which are beneficial to the skin.

12 teaspoon olive oil should be added to the mixture. Olive oil is high in vitamin E, which moisturizes the skin while also fighting free radicals and irritations.

Add three drops of geranium essential oil to the mix. Geranium oil can help to minimize scarring, enhance blood circulation, tone the skin, and encourage the regeneration of new cells. Geranium is derived from the Pelargonium plant, which is commonly used to treat a variety of skin conditions.

Geranium oil has antibacterial, astringent, tonic, and anti-infectious properties.

Add three drops of lavender essential oil to the mix. Lavender oil has a soothing effect on the skin and aids in the reduction of fine lines and wrinkles on the face.

Lavender contains phytochemicals such as linalool and linalyl acetate, which help to promote skin health.

Add 2 tbsp. beeswax to the mix. Anti-inflammatory, antibacterial, and antiviral properties are all provided by beeswax. Beeswax-based creams, lotions, and soaps can significantly alleviate dry, rough skin.

This can help to decrease the effects of aging on the skin, particularly wrinkles.

Add a quarter teaspoon of vitamin E oil to the mix. Vitamin E is an important antioxidant because it protects cell membranes and the enzymes that are involved in them from harm. Vitamin E assists in the inactivation of free radicals, making them less likely to cause harm and slowing the aging of the skin.

Applying vitamin E to the skin can help protect it from the sun's rays while also limiting the creation of cancer-causing cells.

Add 1 tablespoon of shea butter to the mixture. Shea butter is also known as a vitamin A cream that is made entirely of natural ingredients. It's regarded for being a great moisturizer and for fighting dry skin. Shea butter is used as an anti-aging treatment because of its anti-inflammatory and hydrating characteristics.

Inflammation and UV damage are the two main causes of aging.

As a result, vitamin A's damage-reversing capabilities may be advantageous for wrinkle reduction and collagen renewal.

Simmer the mixture after adding all of the oils. Simmer the contents of the glass jar in a pot filled with 3–4 inches (7.6–10.2 cm) of water. To make a smooth and easy-to-apply formulation, fully combine all of the components.

Allow the components to melt in the jar without the lid.

Stir once in a while.

Pour the contents into a small glass jar once it has melted and is properly blended.

Allow it to cool to room temperature before using.

To store your cream, transfer it to an apothecary bottle or keep it in the jar. Transfer the cream to an apothecary bottle or keep it in its jar until it has set. Then store it in the refrigerator.

The vitamin C cream has a two-week shelf life.

To see the results of the vitamin C cream, apply it to your skin. After you've finished making your cream, test it on your skin with a small amount, as some people are allergic to ascorbic acid (Vitamin C).

A Sincere Discussion About Ageing And The Field Of Anti-Aging

Why do so many people fear aging, despite the fact that it is a normal process? When you hear the phrases "growing older" or "old age pensioner," what comes to mind? Is aging, as we know it, unavoidable? It doesn't have to be that way.

Although no magic elixir has yet been discovered, the pursuit of the 'fountain of youth' has absorbed a great deal of energy and inquiry throughout the centuries, and considerable light has been shed on the subject in recent years. We now know there is a lot we can do to slow down the aging process thanks to all of this effort. The way you live can have a big impact on whether the degenerative process is sped up or slowed down.

Of course, aging is unavoidable, but is so much pain as well? Around 85% of diseases are degenerative, with the other 15% being hereditary, infectious, or trauma-related. So, what causes our bodies to deteriorate so quickly? It always makes me wonder why we take better care of our automobiles than we do of ourselves. However, when the old one wears out, we may walk out and get a new one at any moment. It's not as simple for us to exchange our old bodies for new ones. "There are bits we can have replaced," you remark. Yes, there are, including a new hip joint, a new heart or merely the valves, a new liver, or new blood from a transfusion, and many other things.

Returning to our automobile, we don't usually wait for it to break down; instead, we have it maintained on a regular basis to ensure that it has all it requires to do its everyday tasks effectively. The key word here is 'well,' not 'just spluttering a long'. We should treat ourselves with the same respect, providing our bodies with what they require to successfully complete their everyday tasks. The majority of people will wait until their bodies fail.

So, getting back to the point, why do our bodies deteriorate? Researchers have proposed numerous theories, including the Hayflick Limit Theory, which states that each cell has a program that restricts the number of divisions a cell may make before dying. Another idea is the Garbage Accumulation Theory, which states that our cells produce more waste than they are capable of removing, with our regular foods and lifestyles assisting us. The accumulation of waste and toxins in the cell causes the cell to drown in its own poisonous waste.

The other major idea is the free-radical theory, which was first proposed more than 50 years ago and provides an explanation for degenerative disease, accelerated aging, and prevention or, at the very least, delaying its onset until later in life. Free radicals prowl the countryside, attempting to break up stable molecular pairs by taking their companions. It's a little like a bachelor separating happy married couples. When a free radical succeeds in stealing a partner, the other molecule becomes unpaired, unstable, and a free radical on the search, a bachelor. This response is similar to the domino effect, in which a cell-damaging viscous circle sets off a chain reaction.

The oxygen-based free radicals, also known as oxy-radicals, receive the greatest attention. These tiny molecules cause the free-radical damage we call oxidative stress, which contributes to degenerative diseases in the same way that rust does to metal. We may slow down this process by providing a protective coating to the metal, which helps to prevent oxygen and moisture from doing their worst. We can also extend the life of the metal by adding a primer and then a layer of paint. We can extend the life of metal by several years by protecting it from free radicals.

There are things we can do to protect ourselves and slow down the aging process. We may slow down our own rusting, but most individuals opt for a lifestyle that accelerates the process.

Having said that, not all free radicals are toxic; we utilise certain free radical activity to help fight bacterial and viral diseases. These free-radical bachelors are also involved in the creation of important compounds like prostaglandins, which are hormone-like molecules that are essential to numerous bodily activities. Free radicals are also released by our bodies during energy generation, such as during severe exercise, lengthy periods of stress, excitement, rage, or infection.

The vast majority of our oxidative damage in our bodies, however, is caused by excess free radicals present in our environment and the foods we eat, rather than those produced naturally by our own metabolism. Free radicals are formed by air pollution, tobacco smoke, toxic waste, herbicides, pesticides, chemicals in cosmetics or cleaning goods, preservatives, additives in processed meals, and processed oils. When you combine these variables with an abundance of negative thoughts, you have a recipe for premature aging and harm. So, what can we do to safeguard ourselves from this annihilation? What can we do to give our bodies the tools they need to deal with all of this devastation?

Antioxidants, as most of us are aware, prevent or delay the damage produced by free radicals. Our current environment puts a significant amount of stress on our bodies over which we have little control and frequently no choice. We do, however, have the option of consuming anti-oxidants or free radicals, which will immediately speed up or slow down our aging process. Antioxidants are similar to Kamikaze pilots in that they self-sacrifice by donating one of their own electrons. Certain vitamins and minerals, as well as plant chemicals, are powerful anti-oxidants that keep us from rusting. Researchers have repeatedly stated that a lack of antioxidants contributes to age-related degenerative diseases such as heart disease, diabetes, arthritis, vision difficulties, discomfort, and unnecessary suffering.

The idea is to view health care as a means of fostering wellbeing rather than treating illness; the two are not synonymous. Waiting to treat a disease is more difficult and expensive than preventing it. 'I don't want to live to 110,' people frequently tell me in our clinic when addressing lifestyle adjustments. I'm not suggesting that changing your lifestyle will ensure that you live a long life. It's all about the quality of life, and we owe it to ourselves to be as happy and healthy as we possibly can. Maintain a good attitude and take an active role in your own health.

To you, what does prevention imply? When I ask individuals about their health, they always say they are in excellent shape. So, what does it mean to be healthy? Is being healthy just the absence of a certain disease? In other words, because your doctor has not given you a label, such as angina or diabetes, you must be well. I hear comments like, "Every year, I get my annual check-ups and other tests, and I am told I am perfectly OK." What does it imply when it says "100% okay"?

People I see consume and drink a variety of harmful foods and beverages, are inactive, are frequently overweight, and put up with a variety of bodily annoyances. Aches and pains, headaches, migraines, clogged noses, severe digestive problems, asthma, insomnia, exhaustion, and numerous skin issues such as eczema, hypoglycemia, and more are all common complaints. However, they would consider themselves to be in good health. Many people I know regard traditional tests as a "preventative" measure or treatment.

This reminds me of 'Russian roulette,' where you keep pushing the trigger until one day, bang! The tests then come back with a 'negative result' one day out of nowhere—you've taken the bullet! It was as simple as that. Suddenly, you've developed heart disease or diabetes, or your thyroid has ceased functioning correctly. So why should you be concerned if the tests continue to show that you are safe this time, that the barrel was empty this time? In reality, a thyroid problem or a heart condition do not appear out of nowhere. It has taken a very long time to develop. Few tests can detect problems in their early stages, such as a malfunctioning thyroid. The tests will continue to demonstrate that your thyroid is in perfect working order. What happened in the interval, the time leading up to this situation, when you were "broken" and told your thyroid was under-active and you needed medication? Of course, there are circumstances where a thyroid could develop a problem over night, such as in the event of a vehicle accident, where whiplash can have a significant impact on thyroid function.

It's true that some tumors can be discovered in their early stages, which is fantastic. However, most studies consistently suggest that leading a truly healthy lifestyle can reduce our risks of developing cancer in the first place. Furthermore, a typical lifestyle promotes the onset of cancer. For example, you might elect to take 'hormone replacement estrogens' and get an annual mammography as a 'preventative step,' because artificial oestrogen has been linked to an increased risk of breast cancer.

Many women perceive mammograms to be a prophylactic measure, and they wait and see.

To me, prevention means not taking anything that would encourage cancer in the first place, but instead looking for herbs, vitamins, and a change in lifestyle that will help you avoid the natural transition and, in the long run, improve your quality of life.

This is in view of the fact that the menopause is a normal process, despite the fact that it has been labeled as an illness by the medical community. After all, the tests keep telling you that you are 100 percent. Eat, drink, and have a good time.

Or perhaps you believe you are one of the few people who can get away with living a certain way and not pay the price afterwards. Many of the main ailments that plague the developed Western world are actually avoidable through dietary and lifestyle adjustments. Change your lifestyle today, rather than waiting until it's too late (a negative test result). Now is the time to get healthy.

This is where alternative medicine and traditional medicine diverge. We consider health as more than merely the absence of disease; it is a genuine condition of well-being and vitality. We consider all symptoms and indicators to be relevant (no matter how minor) since they all add up to offer a picture of your current health, including which organs and systems are struggling, as well as any shortages or imbalances you may have.

I want to be clear that testing are necessary, but don't be complacent just because your tests show everything is fine. Chronic illnesses take years to develop, and they are often undiscovered until they are far established.

Scientific data supports the premise that the sort of diet we eat has a profound and fundamental impact on how we age, with far more far-reaching repercussions than our inherited DNA. We have no control over our genes, but we do have control over our lifestyles. What exactly does this imply? Several people have told me that they have diabetes relatives. As a result, they believe they have no control over their own fate and that they, too, will become diabetes in the future. Despite this, I watch them consume a lot of refined carbohydrates such as doughnuts, cookies, bread, pancakes, spaghetti, chocolate, sweet meals, drinks, and coffees, with very little fresh food. Their diet is severely deficient in essential nutrients, yet is chock-full of things that hasten aging and induce even more pain. Though this diet does not guarantee diabetes, it does increase your chances of developing the disease, regardless of whether you have close relatives who have diabetes.

Close relatives with diabetes and a similar lifestyle, on the other hand, the odds are very high. A self-fulfilling prophecy, if you will. You not only inherit genes, but also habits. You may have developed a taste for raw seafood if you were born in Japan, and a liking for doughnuts if you were born in America. That is due to acquired taste and habits, not to DNA.

When we think of aging, we usually associate it with some degree of physical and mental decline; yet, many people live long lives with quite good physical and mental health. A healthy life is influenced by a variety of factors, including a person's constitution, family or community, previous lifestyle, and whether they are lonely or fulfilled. Whether they smoke or consume excessive amounts of alcohol. Diet is important for our physical and mental health, but it is not the only factor to consider. There has been just too much research done to deny the idea that aging can be a really pleasurable experience. They have the potential to be the best years of your life. There is a great deal to anticipate.

I recently met a 55-year-old man in our clinic who had mild diabetes, high blood pressure, high cholesterol, poor digestion, heartburn, and was overweight, but his main concern was that he had been denied additional medical insurance (he was from the United States) due to his state of health, the amount of surgery he'd already had, and the large amounts of medication he was taking. In modern Western civilization, this man's situation is fairly common.

On the other hand, there is a 64-year-old man who comes to the clinic for acupuncture as part of his preventative maintenance program, has none of these issues, is not overweight, and is incredibly fit, still riding his bike for miles up and down the mountains around here. For the time being, I'm not expecting you to run out and buy a mountain bike; rather, I'm pointing out that everything is possible; you may choose your course, or course of travel, as it were. The first man has all of the conditions that have been established to be self-inflicted by his lifestyle choices, and that these problems can be improved or even reversed by making the proper choices.

In fact, following treatment, lifestyle adjustments, and supplementation, the first man has achieved significant progress in a variety of areas. His recent blood tests show that his bad cholesterol, triglycerides, blood pressure, and weight had all decreased, as has his medication. He's a completely different person now.

We are everyone at danger of not getting enough nutrients as a result of food refining and processing, but this danger increases as we age due to a loss in our digestive capacity. As a result of a decrease in overall activity, fewer calories are required, and appetite drops, which may be attributable in part to changes in taste and smell. Dehydration is more likely as we age because we lose our sensation of thirst. After years of mistreatment, our digestive system begins to cause us problems. The stomach's production of digestive juices and enzymes slows down, affecting B12, iron, and calcium absorption, to mention a few. Lactase production is decreased, resulting in milk intolerance.

Constipation is a common problem as we age, as we require more fiber than we did when we were younger. Medication can alter how food tastes, produce nausea, or affect how the bowels function. For some of us, simply having to dine alone can discourage us from cooking and eating healthy. Smoking depletes the body of several essential elements. The list of nutrients required to repair joint 'wear and tear,' to maintain healthy bones and teeth is infinite. Drink in moderation; more than a modest amount of alcohol can be harmful to your overall health and well-being. Are your tests revealing high blood pressure and cholesterol levels, and the scales proclaiming "you are overweight," but you already knew this because your "lower front" was causing your "lower back" to suffer? They are informing you that you are now diabetic. That menopause is a medical condition! What does this mean when it comes to puberty? It's only a matter of time before you develop osteoporosis. No man is immune to prostate cancer! Those incontinence pads are meant to be used for the rest of your life! And before you know it, you'll be fighting with fake teeth!

We rarely bat an eyelid in our culture when we hear of someone suffering from diabetes, stroke, arthritis, or heart disease after a certain age (though now at a younger age than before). However, if we lived in a more conventional society, these diseases would be quite rare at any age, but especially so at such a young age as we are now experiencing them, and they would be quite a topic of conversation

Women who consume a traditional Japanese diet, for example, rarely get osteoporosis and have few menopause symptoms. Despite this, the modern Japanese lady who eats a standard western diet suffers from osteoporosis and menopause symptoms! This isn't due to genetics.

We must examine the facts: a rapid decrease is not unavoidable. There is a lot of research that shows that things can change, that your life can change. That your life can be so much better later in life; you can be healthier, happier, leaner, and more active. Do not be brainwashed by advertising corporations, or by the allure of addictive chemicals on store shelves that age you.

It's never too early or too late to begin an anti-aging regimen, so think positively.

The Natural Solutions

The majority of anti-aging products on the market are intended to improve the appearance of the skin and hair. This is because the majority of people believe "anti-aging remedies" are meant to make you seem younger. The aging process, on the other hand, is far more sophisticated than what happens to your body on the surface. It also has to do with what's going on inside your body. Hormonal balance, immune system strength, mental capacity, sex drive, feeling of balance, movement, stamina, joint discomfort, and other factors can all be affected by aging. The following are 12 natural anti-aging remedies that will help you slow down the aging process on the inside and out:

1. Increase Your Water Consumption

The simplest thing you can do to slow down the aging process is to drink more water. According to studies, the majority of people are chronically dehydrated. Water lubricates the skin from the inside out and is considerably superior to any moisturizer available. Water also aids in the elasticity of the skin. This indicates that the more water you drink, the less wrinkled and smoother your skin will be.

2. Consume More Blueberries and Antioxidant-Rich Foods

Who needs anti-aging cosmetics when eating antioxidants can provide a much larger anti-aging benefit? Antioxidants protect the body from free radicals, which generate at an increasing rate as we age. You'll eliminate more free radicals if you eat more antioxidants. Unfortunately, natural antioxidants are in short supply in today's diet. The majority of antioxidants have been removed from processed foods, which have become a staple in the American diet.

Antioxidants can be obtained by eating a wide variety of fresh fruits and vegetables, particularly organic ones. Antioxidants abound in blueberries in particular. Other berries, such as raspberries, strawberries, and blackberries, are similarly high in antioxidants.

3. Eat a Magnesium-Rich Diet

Men and women should take between 300 and 400 mg of magnesium each day, according to the National Institutes of Health (NIH). However, research have shown that the majority of people do not consume this amount. This is due to the fact that most of us do not consume enough magnesium-rich meals. Dark leafy greens like spinach, kale, and mustard greens are examples of these foods. Green herbs including parsley, cilantro, basil, thyme, and dill are also included. Magnesium is also abundant in nuts and whole grains.

Magnesium aids in the regulation of blood sugar levels through regulating insulin levels in the body. Maintaining a healthy blood sugar level helps to prevent glycation, which is one of the main causes of aging.

Sugar degrades and deforms protein during glycation.

4. Eat the Right Foods to Reduce Inflammation Chronic inflammation worsens as people get older.

When the inflammatory process is increased, it causes premature aging. Reduced inflammation, on the other hand, can help to slow down the aging process. The skin wrinkles as a result of inflammation. Chronic inflammation also contributes to other signs of aging, such as a loss of mental capability and physical stiffness.

5. Workout

Exercise is one of the most effective strategies to minimize cellulite. Squats and lunges are two exercises that can help you get rid of cellulite in your thighs. Sagging skin is also prevented by weight training.

Tightening the muscles in the face might assist to keep the skin on the face from drooping. Aerobic exercise can also aid to slow down the aging process in general. This form of exercise enhances the immune system and improves the efficiency of all of your body's organs. Organs like the liver and kidneys, which are crucial to the detoxification process, are included.

6. Put an end to the yo-yo diet

The connective tissue between the skin and the muscles stretches when you enter into the vicious cycle of losing weight and then gaining it back. The skin sags as a result of this. If you need to reduce weight, it is far better to do it slowly and steadily and then maintain your weight loss.

7. Reduce Your Anxiety

It's no coincidence that our presidents all appear to be getting older while in office. Being president is a very difficult job, and stress accelerates the aging process more than anything else. Stress disrupts the body's hormone balance, shortens cell lifespan, causes wrinkles and hair loss, modifies DNA to make it difficult to replicate, and produces high levels of the hormone cortisol, which speeds up the aging process.

You must find techniques to reduce your stress levels if you want to live longer and slow down the aging process.

The first step is to assess your situation and identify your primary and secondary stressors.

Next, if it is practicable, eliminate or lessen stress. Finally, find ways to relax and de-stress.

Relaxation techniques include exercise, yoga, long walks, writing, listening to music, and aromatherapy. Examine your options to see what works best for you. The most important thing is to recognize the need for it and to make sure you can fit it into your schedule.

8. Gain a better understanding of how to deal with stress

Some people find it beneficial to keep a temporary diary of items that cause stress. Once you've figured out what's causing the tension, it'll be much easier to stop it before it gets out of hand. It also provides you the much-needed permission to treat yourself to something lovely to relieve stress. You could, for example, plan a relaxing massage and/or delegate additional responsibilities to your partner.

9. Use sunscreen to protect your skin from the sun.

When it comes to wrinkles, most people are facing an uphill battle by the time they reach their thirties. Putting too much pressure on the skin is counterproductive. UV radiation creates wrinkles and black patches on the skin, as well as malignant growth. UV damages collagen and stops it from being produced by the body. It is critical to wear a broad spectrum SPF 30 sunscreen when exposed to the sun. This will aid in the prevention of dark sun spots from forming, as well as the darkening of existing dark spots. Wearing protective apparel, such as a wide-brimmed hat, is also an option.

10. Detoxification Of The Body

Heavy metals and other environmental toxins hasten the aging process while also causing other health problems. Three to four times a year, you should detox to keep them out of your system. Drinking more water aids in the detoxification of the body. Eating extra greens can also help the body detox. Two meals are even more beneficial. Spirulina, blue - green algae, and Chorella, green algae are examples. When you're trying to detox, a teaspoon to three teaspoons of supercharged algae mixed in water is an excellent way to start the day.

Making a tea with fresh parsley or cilantro is also a fantastic way to detox.

11. Increase your sleep time

The body regenerates itself as you sleep. While we sleep, our cells rebuild themselves more quickly. Nutrients are better absorbed. As we sleep, our cortisol levels naturally decrease. Dreaming aids in the organization of our thoughts, which can help with memory problems.

12. Don't Smoke

Smoking hastens the aging process. It wreaks havoc on the skin's collagen and elastin layers. The skin becomes less elastic and wrinkles more as a result of this. Smoking also decreases blood flow and oxygenation to cells, resulting in skin damage. If you smoke, you must quit as soon as possible, regardless of how difficult it may be.

To summarize, each of these natural anti-aging therapies is effective, but you shouldn't anticipate a miracle from any of them. However, when many natural methods are combined, the result can be rather stunning. The elusive fountain of youth is a mosaic of good living rather than a single source.

Formulas for Prevent Aging Knees

Over time, aging knees can have a negative impact on both your physical ability and your self-image. When your knees lose movement, it affects your physical well-being, typically resulting in pain and suffering.

Some folks are also concerned about how their knees will age. Both of these issues with aging knees can be avoided with a few lifestyle modifications and a long-term commitment to improving overall knee health.

Formula One: How to Avoid Knee Injuries

1. Use kneepads.

If you're participating in an activity that could hurt your knees, such as a sport that requires you to fall, you should safeguard them first. If you're doing anything that could result in a fall or pressure on your knees, you should wear knee pads.

Volleyball players, for example, should wear knee pads to protect their knees when falling or diving for the ball.

Knee pads can be useful for a variety of activities other than sports. Wear knee pads or use a cushioned pad to kneel on when you are on your knees, for example, if you spend a lot of time weeding in your yard.

2. Don't do anything that could hurt your knees.

Certain types of motions can put a lot of strain on your knees. The knee can be strained and injured by sudden movements or direct pressure on the front or rear of the knee. This is especially true if you already have a knee injury or disease, such as osteoarthritis.

This indicates you should exercise caution when lifting large items. Make sure you don't spin while lifting, as this puts your knee under unnaturally high pressure.

Also, avoid bending your knees to the point where they are overextended. When exercising, for example, be particular careful not to overextend your knees.

3. Maintain a healthy weight.

Excessive weight on the knees might cause them to age prematurely. Maintain a healthy weight to keep your knees from becoming painful and damaged.

Losing weight reduces the amount of stress on your knees. Your knees will likely operate considerably better over time if you can reduce that stress.

4. Eat a diet that is low in inflammation.

It's a good idea to consume an anti-inflammatory diet for healthy joint health. The goal of this diet is to eat foods that lower inflammation while avoiding those that cause inflammation.

Fish, green vegetables, olive oil, fruit, and nuts are all anti-inflammatory foods.

Fried meals, drink, refined carbohydrates, fat, and processed meats are all pro-inflammatory foods.

5. Inquire about drugs and other therapies with your doctor.

Consult your doctor if your knees are bothering you or if you are concerned about developing problems with them in the future. There are many things you can do to protect and enhance the health of your knees, as well as ease pain. Among the possibilities are:

Using a knee brace to maintain your knee aligned properly.

Injections of cortisone to relieve pain and inflammation in the knees.

Acetaminophen or ibuprofen are examples of over-the-counter pain relievers.

Knee surgery is used to treat severe or persistent knee discomfort.

Formula Two: Performing Knee-Friendly Exercises

1. Exercise should be preceded by a warm-up.

Warming up your knees will prepare them for action and lessen the risk of damage. Stretch the muscles in your thighs to adequately warm up your knees. These stretches will warm up your knees as well.

Quad stretches, walking lunges, and hamstring stretches, for example, are all ideal knee warm-ups.

2. Weight train with a specific goal in mind.

You can improve the function of your joints and minimize the pressure on them by strengthening the muscles that surround them. The following muscles should be targeted in your workout:

Quadriceps is a muscle group that consists of four muscles. The muscles on the front of your thigh are known as quadriceps. Lunges and leg extensions can be used to target these muscles.

Hamstrings are the muscles in the back of the legs. The muscles in the back of your thighs are called quadriceps. Leg curls and squats might help you target these muscles.

Abductors are people who kidnap others. These are located on the outside of your thigh. Side-lying leg lifts or an abductor machine at the gym can help you target these muscles.

Adductors are a type of adductor. The muscles on the inner of your thighs are used for this. Holding an exercise ball between your feet with your legs in the air or utilizing an adductor machine at the gym can help you target these muscles.

Gluteals are a kind of glutamate. These are the muscles in your buttocks. Squats, lunges, and donkey kicks can help to improve these muscles.

3. Make your knees more flexible.

The correct types of exercise can help you maintain knee flexibility and avoid age-related wear and strain. Spend some of your training time focusing on flexibility to keep your knees from aging prematurely. Swimming and yoga, for example, are low-impact exercises that can help keep your knees in good form over time.

Your joints may become less flexible as you age. Stretching them on a regular basis can assist you avoid losing them.

4. Exercises with a high impact should be avoided.

While it is important to exercise your knees, if done incorrectly, some exercises might cause more harm than good. Running and other high-impact exercises, such as those that demand a lot of jumping, in particular, can put a lot of strain on your knees. Do these types of exercises on soft surfaces or in well-cushioned, well-fitting shoes to reduce the impact. It's a good idea to do everything you can to reduce the impact of high-impact activity.

Try to exercise in methods that are gentler on your joints, such as swimming, riding, or walking on a low or no-resistance elliptical walker.

Running may be beneficial to your knees, according to some data. Recent scientific studies reveal that runners are less prone than non-runners to have knee problems, however this could be due to the fact that runners are more likely to carry less weight on their bodies.

Formula Three: Preventing Wrinkled and Saggy Knees

1. Make use of skin care products.

To produce smooth and tight skin on the knees, a range of skin treatments can be used. Acid treatments to remove dead and damaged skin, as well as moisturizing treatments to keep skin smooth and elastic throughout time, are among these options.

An alpha hydroxy acid treatment on the knees and elbows can be highly successful in removing old and dried up skin. These products are available over the counter and should be used according to the instructions on the package.

2. Focus on certain workouts.

Exercising your leg muscles might result in increased skin tension across your legs. Your skin will be better supported and the areas around your knees should stiffen up as your muscle mass increases.

Spend some time throughout your everyday workout, for example, working on your quadriceps. Pumping these muscles, which are placed right above your knees, should also tighten the skin on your knee.

3. Use weight-loss methods that are gradual.

When you lose a lot of weight all at once, you can end up with a lot of saggy skin all over your body. The appearance of your knees may be affected by this sagginess.

Rather of embarking on a crash diet, aim to lose a pound or two a week so your skin can catch up and tighten on its own.

However, if you're losing a lot of weight, your body may not be able to absorb all of the skin. The excess skin will not always tighten on its own in situations like this.

4. Think about cosmetic surgery.

If you are self-conscious about the appearance of your knees, surgery is a possibility. Liposuction and lasers are used by plastic surgeons to minimize the amount of loose skin and fat on your knee, resulting in tighter skin.

Plastic surgery, unlike the other alternatives for avoiding aging knees, comes with some health hazards. Before having this medical procedure, talk to your doctor about the probable dangers of anesthesia and surgery.

In conclusion, it is my strong believe that this book has expanded your knowledge on the best ways to live an amazing life and reverse or halt the aging process through diets.

Now go out there, be positive, and put into practice all that I have shared with you.